Zahra Sarafraz
Seyyed Ali Musavi
Mohammad Hossein Azaraein

Rare Parotid Gland Neoplasms

AF153284

Zahra Sarafraz
Seyyed Ali Musavi
Mohammad Hossein Azaraein

Rare Parotid Gland Neoplasms

Diagnosis,Management and review of literatures

LAP LAMBERT Academic Publishing

Impressum / Imprint

Bibliografische Information der Deutschen Nationalbibliothek: Die Deutsche Nationalbibliothek verzeichnet diese Publikation in der Deutschen Nationalbibliografie; detaillierte bibliografische Daten sind im Internet über http://dnb.d-nb.de abrufbar.
Alle in diesem Buch genannten Marken und Produktnamen unterliegen warenzeichen-, marken- oder patentrechtlichem Schutz bzw. sind Warenzeichen oder eingetragene Warenzeichen der jeweiligen Inhaber. Die Wiedergabe von Marken, Produktnamen, Gebrauchsnamen, Handelsnamen, Warenbezeichnungen u.s.w. in diesem Werk berechtigt auch ohne besondere Kennzeichnung nicht zu der Annahme, dass solche Namen im Sinne der Warenzeichen- und Markenschutzgesetzgebung als frei zu betrachten wären und daher von jedermann benutzt werden dürften.

Bibliographic information published by the Deutsche Nationalbibliothek: The Deutsche Nationalbibliothek lists this publication in the Deutsche Nationalbibliografie; detailed bibliographic data are available in the Internet at http://dnb.d-nb.de.
Any brand names and product names mentioned in this book are subject to trademark, brand or patent protection and are trademarks or registered trademarks of their respective holders. The use of brand names, product names, common names, trade names, product descriptions etc. even without a particular marking in this work is in no way to be construed to mean that such names may be regarded as unrestricted in respect of trademark and brand protection legislation and could thus be used by anyone.

Coverbild / Cover image: www.ingimage.com

Verlag / Publisher:
LAP LAMBERT Academic Publishing
ist ein Imprint der / is a trademark of
OmniScriptum GmbH & Co. KG
Heinrich-Böcking-Str. 6-8, 66121 Saarbrücken, Deutschland / Germany
Email: info@lap-publishing.com

Herstellung: siehe letzte Seite /
Printed at: see last page
ISBN: 978-3-659-70503-8

Rare Parotid Gland Neoplasms

Contents

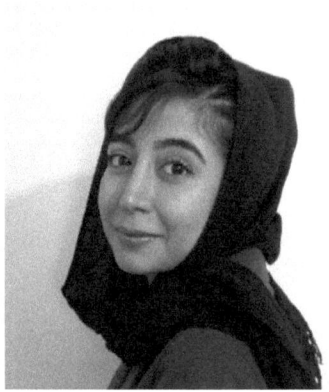

Preface

Although parotid gland cancer is relatively rare, it still constitutes as a serious health problem among population because of its poor prognosis, distant metastases and possibility of facial nerve weakness due to tumor invasion or iatrogenic events. Twenty percent of all patients will develop distant metastases despite its large variety of histologic types. Patients with high-grade tumors have a higher chance of developing distant metastases than those with lower-grade tumors. But for low grade and benign tumors there are other concepts such as error in histologic diagnosis and inadequate management.

This paper is composed of five parts. In each part at first we present rare parotid gland entity then we investigate the problem in form of case report and study their imaging, laboratory tests, differential diagnosis and treatment with follow up status. At the end we discuss about their management with review of literatures.

Dr. Zahra Sarafraz

Otolaryngologist, Department of Otolaryngology,
Faculty of Medicine and Health Sciences,
Yazd University of Medical Sciences, Yazd, Iran
E-mail: zahra.sarafraz@yahoo.com
Tel: +98.9125071121

Contributors

Zahra Sarafraz, MD
Otolaryngologist, Unit of Otolaryngology Medicine, Department of Otolaryngology, Faculty of Medicine and Health Sciences, Yazd University of Medical Sciences, Yazd, Iran

Mohammad Hossein Azaraein, MD
Student research committee, Unit of Otolaryngology Medicine, Department of Otolaryngology, Faculty of Medicine and Health Sciences, Yazd University of Medical Sciences, Yazd, Iran

Seyyed Ali Musavi, MD
Assistant professor, Unit of Otolaryngology Medicine, Department of Otolaryngology, Faculty of Medicine and Health Sciences, Yazd University of Medical Sciences, Yazd, Iran

Corresponding author:
Zahra Sarafraz, Otolaryngologist,
Unit of Otolaryngology Medicine, Department of Otolaryngology,
Faculty of Medicine and Health Sciences,
Yazd University of Medical Sciences, Yazd, Iran

Acknowledgements
The authors gratefully acknowledge Dr. Mansour Moghimi and Dr. Fariba Binesh who helped us for structural and scientific editing of this paper.

Rare Parotid Gland Neoplasms

Part 1

Basal Cell Adenocarcinoma

Basal Cell Adenocarcinoma (BCAC) is one of the rare subtypes of carcinoma of salivary glands. It is a salivary gland malignancy that was first recognized as a distinct neoplastic entity in World Health Organization's (WHO's) classification of salivary gland tumors in 1991. BCAC of the salivary gland is a rare neoplasm, especially in the parotid gland. It composes 1.6% of all salivary gland neoplasms and 2.9% of malignant salivary gland neoplasms. The most important differential diagnosis of BCAC is Basal Cell Adenoma (BCA), but the behavior of BCAC is invasive and destructive with perineural and vascular invasion [1, 2]. The histopathology of BCAC shows two cell types, i.e., small basaloid epithelial cells at the periphery and larger epithelial cells in the center of the tumour clusters .Most cases of BCAC are de novo, but 25% of BCACs originate from pre-existing basal cell adenomas. In general, BCAC has a good prognosis. Metastasis is rare but may recur locally [3, 4]. BCACs are categorized into four types on the basis of their growth patterns, i.e., solid, trabecular, tubular, and membranous; the solid type is the most common [2, 5]. In this part we discuss BCAC in 71-year-old patient with some interesting features that were different from those in previous case reports.

I. Basal Cell Adenocarcinoma of the Parotid Gland in an Elderly Iranian Woman and Review of the Literature

Abstract

Basal Cell Adenocarcinoma (BCAC) is a rare subtype of carcinoma of salivary glands. It accounts for 1.6% of all salivary gland neoplasms and 2.9% of malignant salivary gland neoplasms. BCAC is especially rare in parotid glands. The biological behavior of BCAC is invasive and destructive, with perineural and vascular invasion. This paper presents a BCAC with multiple recurrences and wide local extension in a 71-year-old Iranian woman with a 30-year history of a large mass on the right side of her neck. The importance aspects of this case were its long duration, multiple recurrences, facial nerve involvement and the use of clinicopathological criteria for diagnosis.

Keywords: Basal cell Adenocarcinoma, parotid gland, neoplasm

Case Presentation

A 71-year-old Iranian woman with a 30-year history of a large mass on the right side of her neck was referred to the Otolaryngology Department at Shahid Sadoughi Hospital in Yazd, Iran in 2012. She presented with a firm, fixed, non-tender mass on the right side of her neck that measured 10×15 cm with normal skin with no apparent invasion. The clinical examination provided no evidence of cervical lymphadenopathy. The patient complained about mild dysphagia, and the oropharyngeal exam revealed a bulging mass in the right side of the oral cavity. Facial movements were partially asymmetrical on the right side of the lower lip (other branches of facial nerve were intact).

Also, a bulge was found on the anterior wall of the right external auditory canal. A superficial parotidectomy was performed 10 years ago; subsequently, the patient experienced five recurrences of masses on her neck, and the last recurrence occurred four years ago. Unfortunately, we don't have any documented pathology from her previous surgeries. An investigation of the patients' family history showed no occurrence of cancer.

Investigation

Imaging

Abdominal ultrasonography revealed no abnormality, and the chest X-ray indicated no signs of metastasis. The CT scan showed a large, irregular mass in the right parotid gland, bulging into the parapharyngeal space. It extended up to the base of the skull (Figure1).

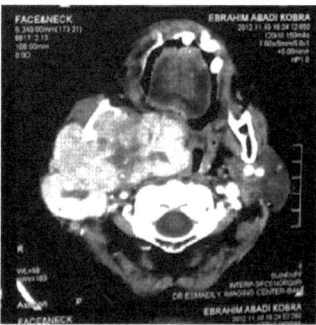

Figure 1: Mass extension in patient axial cut of neck CT scan

Histopathology and other laboratory findings

In the gross pathological examination, the tumour had creamy colored nodular tissue that measured 16×14×5 cm with firm consistency and lobular appearance in the cut section. Some of nodules had thin capsules with calcified foci. Microscopic examination revealed a tumoural lesion with a multinodular pattern composed of basaloid cells that had round-to-oval nuclei with fine nucleoli and scant-to-moderate cytoplasm. Cells arranged in lobules, sheets, aggregates cords, trabeculae and membranous pattern. Hyaline Periodic Acid Schiff (PAS) positive materials with palisading and jigsaw puzzle patterns were observed. There were no more than six mitoses in the 10 High Power Field (HPF).

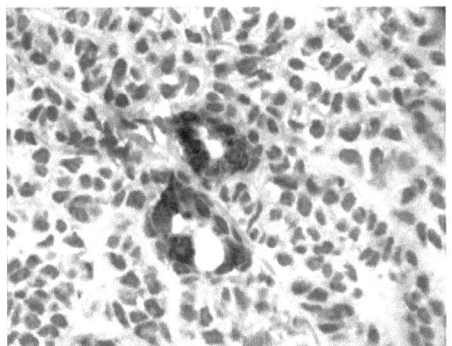

Figure2. EMA immunostaining positive in luminal cell in areas of ductal differentiation

Cellular pleomorphism, necrosis, vascular and perineural invasion, and lymph node metastasis were absent. The primary diagnosis was low-grade basal cell adenocarcinoma. For ruling out other differential diagnoses, Immunohistochemistry (IHC) was performed. The tumoral cells were positive for CK AE1/3, SMA, S100 (moderately positive), EMA and CD117 (positive in luminal cells in areas of ductal differentiation), Vimentin (focally positive), and Ki67 (in 5 to 10% of the tumoral cells). CEA and GFAP were negative (Figures 2 and 3) (Table1).

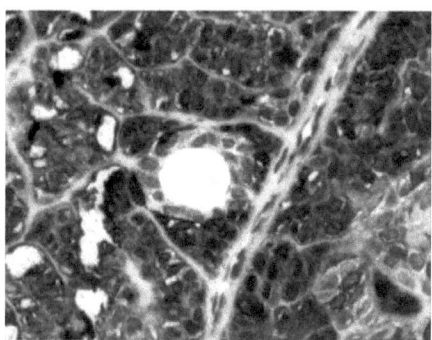

Figure3. ASMA immunostaining positive in abluminal cells.

Antibodies	clone	class	code	Antigen unmasking methods: Microwave retrieval	Dilution
Monoclonal Mouse Anti-Human Smooth Muscle Actin (SMA)	1A4	IG2a, kappa	M0851	15 minutes heating – induced epitope retrieval (750 W) in 10 mmol/L citrate buffer, pH 6	1:75 in 0.02 M PBS, pH 7.2–7.6
Monoclonal Mouse Anti- Human Cytokeratin AE1/AE3	AE1 and AE3	AE1: IgG1, kappa; AE3: IgG1, kappa	M3515	15 minutes heating – induced epitope retrieval (750 W) in 10 mmol/L citrate buffer, pH 6	1:50 in 0.02 M PBS, pH 7.2–7.6
Polyclonal rabbit Anti-S 100	-	-	Z0311 Ig fraction	15 minutes heating – induced epitope retrieval (750 W) in 10 mmol/L citrate buffer, pH 6	1: 300 in 0.02 M PBS, pH 7.2–7.6
Polyclonal Rabbit Anti-Human Carcinoembryonic Antigen (CEA)	-	-	A0115 Ig fraction	15 minutes heating – induced epitope retrieval (750 W) in 10 mmol/L citrate buffer, pH 6	1:100 in 0.02 M PBS, pH 7.2–7.6
Monoclonal Mouse Anti-Human Vimentin (VIM)	V9	IgG1, kappa	M0725 Culture supernatant	15 minutes heating – induced epitope retrieval (750 W) in 10 mmol/L citrate buffer, pH 6	1:30 in 0.02 M PBS, pH 7.2–7.6
Polyclonal Rabbit Anti-Glial Fibrillary Acidic protein (GFAP)	-	-	IS524	15 minutes heating – induced epitope retrieval (750 W) in 10 mmol/L citrate buffer, pH 6	1:30 in 0.02 M PBS, pH 7.2–7.6

Table1. Antibodies used in the immunohistochemical investigation of BCAC

Treatment

The tumor at the base of the skull and the deep portion of the parotid gland were resected, and suprahyoid dissection of the lymph nodes was performed, including the submandibular, submental, and upper third of the jugulodigastric nodes. Except marginal mandibular branch the facial nerve was preserved and post-operative irradiation were conducted.

Outcome and follow-up

At the one-year follow up, she had no recurrence of any of the features associated with BCAC. Also, the metastasis workup revealed no sign of metastasis.

Differential Diagnosis of Salivary Gland Basaloid Lesions

• Basal cell adenoma
• Basal cell adenocarcinoma
• Adenoid cystic carcinoma (solid)
• Cellular pleomorphic adenoma
• Chronic sialadenitis
• Cutaneous basal cell carcinoma
• Metastatic basaloid squamous carcinoma

It is important to be cautious when diagnosing a basal cell tumor because basal cell adenocarcinoma is a low-grade malignancy with an acceptable prognosis, while adenoid cystic carcinoma is an aggressive cancer that requires a more extensive surgical approach (Table2).

Cytologic Features	Basal Cell Adenocarcinoma	Basal Cell Adenoma	Pleomorphic Adenoma	Adenoid Cystic Carcinoma	Chronic Sialadenitis
Cytoarchitecture	Cohesive clusters; haphazard; peripheral palisading; squamous morules	Cohesive clusters; haphazard; peripheral palisading; squamous morules	Single cells and groups; haphazard; ductal structures	3-D cylinders and branching groups; mosaic pattern	Small angulated groups
Cells	Two basaloid cell types	Two basaloid cell types	Often myoepithelial predominant + cuboidal cells	Basaloid cells and variable numbers of myoepithelial cells	Low-cuboidal ductal cells, sparse cellularity
Nuclei	Round to oval; Dark; bland	Round to oval; dark; bland	Round to oval with fine chromatin	Oval to angulated; mild to moderate atypia	Round to oval; dark; bland
Stroma	Intercellular matrix globules; peripheral acellular matrix ribbons	Intercellular matrix globules; peripheral acellular matrix ribbons	Fibrillar myxoid matrix; frayed edges; embedded cells;	Branching tubules and spheres; acellular; sharp borders	Absent
Back ground	Clean with occasional stripped nuclei	Clean with occasional stripped nuclei	Single myoepithelial cells	Clean with occasional stripped nuclei	Mild chronic inflammation

Table2. Cytologic differential diagnosis of selected basaloid lesions.

Discussion

BCAC is slow-growing, locally-destructive tumor. It was first defined as a malignant tumor of the salivary gland in 1991 (1). The most important differential diagnosis for BCAC is basal cell adenoma (1). Both of them have similar histological appearances (basaloid pattern), but infiltrative growth is the distinguishing feature of BCAC. Pathological criteria for the diagnosis of BCAC include infiltrative growth with vascular or perineural invasion. Other features may include nuclear pleomorphism, necrosis, and mitotic activity (3, 4). In our patient, there were no more than six mitoses inthe 10 HPF. Cellular pleomorphism, necrosis, vascular and perineural invasion, and lymph-node metastasis were absent, but, clinically, it was a huge mass (10 x 15 cm) with wide extention and a history of multiple recurrences. Its invasion of the adjacent soft tissues was obvious during surgery. IHC suggested BCAC and ruled out a differential diagnosis. We believe that the diagnosis of BCAC is clinicopathological, and sometimes it is very difficult to distinguish it from basal cell adenoma using only pathological criteria. The rate of metastasis is low, but the rate of local recurrence is high. Metastasis occurs in less than 10% of cases, and only one case involving the lung has been reported (3, 4). Because of their biological behavior and their prognosis, BCACs should be classified as low-grade carcinomas. In our patient, a complete metastasis workup was performed, and there were no features of metastasis. There have been a few descriptions of facial paralysis or additional destruction of the salivary gland, but interesting findings in our patient's case were that the buccal branch of the facial nerve was weak and that the BCAC extended up to the base of the skull, bulging into the parapharyngeal space. Many patients with BCAC recognized after 7-10 years (5), but our patient had it for the long duration of about 30 years with five recurrences. Most patients present with a solitary firm nodule between 1 and 3 cm that is slowly enlarging. The largest tumor described by Ellis et al. was 4 cm

(6), but our patient's tumor was about10 x 15 cm. Local recurrence occurs in about one-third of the cases (5), and our patient had five recurrences over a 30-year period. Our case was unique with respect to its duration, the number of recurrences, and the size of the mass.

BCAC has four subtypes, i.e., solid, membranous, trabecular, and tubular. The solid areas of BCACs are composed of nonluminal cells, some of which contain tonofilaments and well-formed desmosomes; tubulo-trabecular differentiated into both luminal and nonluminal cells. Both growth patterns were associated with the formation of excess basal lamina, marginally and between nonluminal cells. The majority of these tumors are solid. They are characterized by islands and masses within the fibrous connective tissue stroma (5), the histological type of our patients BCAC was membranous. The membranous type is actually the second most frequently-occurring type of BCAC, accounting for about 20% of all occurrences (2). This type has thick, eosinophilic, periodic acid Schiff positive hyaline laminae that surround and separate one tumor nest from another and a jigsaw puzzle formation (Figure4). The trabecular type of BCAC has anastomosing cords of basaloid epithelial cells that look like Chinese characters (2, 5). Muller & Barnes conducted an extensive literature search in 1996, and they concluded that parotid is the most common salivary gland that is involved with BCAC (89% in the parotid, 10% in the submandibular gland, and 1% among the minor salivary glands) (7). In our case, the parotid gland was involved. Most studies recommend wide local excision. Treatment for regional metastasis (neck) is done for significant lymphadenopathy on clinical or radiologic examination, and postoperative radiation is recommended for close surgical margins or following surgical excision of recurrent tumor (7-9).

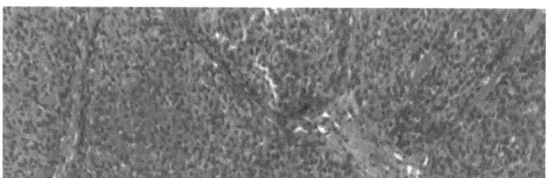

Figure4. Lobules with jigsaw puzzle like pattern in Membranous BCAC

The surgical procedure we performed was resection of the tumor at the base of the skull with deep portion resection of the parotid gland with preservation of the facial nerve. At last we summarise at least 46 cases of parotid gland BCAC from 1990-2014 in two tables and compare them with our case (Tables 3and 4).

Studies	Ellis GL et al 1990	Muller S et al 1996	Kwang II 1997	Ikeda K 1998	Golz A. et al 2000
Cases & Sex	29	7(6 female&1 male)	1(female)	1(female)	1(male)
Age	Adults with Peak incidence 6th decade	46-74	33	73	24
Location	Major salivary glands	Parotid gland(Except one case)	Left Parotid	Right Parotid	Left parotid
Size(mm)	Variable	Variable	20	50	30
common Histologic type	Solid	-	tubulotrabecular type	Solid& Tubular	
Manifestation	-	Parotid mass	Infraauricular mass	Parotid mass	Retroauricular abscess
Facial nerve status	-	Intact	Intact	Intact	Intact
Cervical lymphadenopathy	2	none	Negative	Negative	Negative
Local recurrences	7	2	Negative	Negative	Negative
Distant metastasis	1	1	Negative	Negative	Negative
Site of metastasis	Lung	-	-	-	-
Treatment	Parotidectomy	Local excision	Parotidectomy	Parotidectomy	Total Parotidectomy
Follow up duration	Few months	30 month	24 months	24 Months	30 months
Status after follow up	One case died	Tumor free	Tumor free	Tumor free	Tumor free

Table 3.Review of the literature

Studies	Keiichi Jingu 2010	Mari ML et al 2010	Michael H. Elvey 2011	Hamamoto M 2012	Sarafraz Z. et al 2014
Cases& Sex	4(2 female& 2male)	1(male)	1(male)	1(female)	1(female)
Age	37-81	60	67	58	71
Location	3 cases right and 1 case in left Parotid gland	Bilateral Parotid glands	Parotid	Right parotid	Right parotid
Size(mm)	19-54mm	Right:10mm Left:6mm	-	-	150mm
Dominant Histologic type	-	Tubular	Solid	-	Membranous
Manifestation	Buccal swelling	Incidental in ultrasonography	Parotid mass Pain& swelling In his hand	Parotid mass	Parotid mass
Facial nerve status	Intact	Intact	Intact	Intact	Weakness in buccal branch
Cervical lymphadenopathy	1	Negative	Negative	Negative	Negative
Local recurrences	1	Negative	Negative	Negative	Negative
Distant metastasis	none	Negative	+	Negative	Negative
Site of metastasis	-	-	Second to 5th metacarpal	-	-
Treatment	Parotidectomy +radiotherapy	Parotidectomy	Parotidectomy +radiotherapy Distal forearm amputation	Superficial Parotidectomy +radiotherapy	Parotidectomy +radiotherapy
Follow up duration	3 Months	-	24 months	8 months	48 months
Status after follow up	No recurrence	-	No evidence of metastasis	Tumor free	No recurrence

Table 4.Review of the literature

References
1. Quddus MR, Henley JD, Affify AM, Dardick I, Gnepp DR (1999) Basal cell adenocarcinoma of the salivary gland: an ultrastructural and immunohistochemical study. Oral Surg Oral Med Oral Pathol Oral Radiol Endod 87: 485-492.
2. Sharma R, Saxena S, Bansal R (2007) Basal cell adenocarcinoma: Report of a case affecting the submandibular gland 11: 56-9.
3. Markkanen-Leppanen M, Makitie AA, Passador-Santos F, Leivo I, Hagström J (2010) Bilateral Basal cell adenocarcinoma of the parotid gland: in a recipient of kidney transplant. Clin Med Insights Pathol 3: 1-5.
4. Ward BK, Seethala RR, Barnes EL, Lai SY (2009) Basal cell adenocarcinoma of a hard palate minor salivary gland: case report and review of the literature. Head Neck Oncol 1: 41.
5. Ellis GL, Wiscovitch JG (1990) Basal cell adenocarcinomas of the major salivary glands. Oral Surg Oral Med Oral Pathol 69: 461-469.
6. Hirsch DL, Miles C, Dierks E (2007) Basal cell adenocarcinoma of the parotid gland: report of a case and review of the literature. J Oral Maxillofac Surg 65: 2385-2388.
7. Jayakrishnan A, Elmalah I, Hussain K, Odell EW (2003) Basal cell adenocarcinoma in minor salivary glands. Histopathology 42: 610-614.
8. Yu GY, Ubmuller J, Donath K (1998) Membranous basal cell adenoma of the salivary gland: a clinicopathologic study of 12 cases. Acta Otolaryngol 118: 588-593.
9. Parashar P, Baron E, Papadimitriou JC, Ord RA, Nikitakis NG (2007) Basal cell adenocarcinoma of the oral minor salivary glands: review of the literature and presentation of two cases. Oral Surg Oral Med Oral Pathol Oral Radiol Endod 103: 77-84.
10. Muller S, Barnes L (1996) Basal cell adenocarcinoma of the salivary glands. Report of seven cases and review of the literature. Cancer 78:2471-2477.
11. Kim KI, Oh HE, Mun JS, Kim CH, Choi JS (1997) Basal cell adenocarcinoma of the salivary gland--a case report. J Korean Med Sci12: 461-464.
12. Ikeda K, Watanabe M, Oshima T, Nakabayashi S, Kudo T, et al. (1998) A case of basal cell adenocarcinoma of the parotid gland. Tohoku J Exp Med 186: 51-59.
13. Golz A, Goldenberg D, Ben-Arie Y, Keren R, Netzer A, et al. (2000) Basal cell adenocarcinoma of the parotid gland presenting as a retroauricular abscess. Am J Otolaryngol 21: 421-426.
14. Jingu K, Hasegawa A, Mizo JE, Bessho H, Morikawa T, et al. (2010) Carbon ion radiotherapy for basal cell adenocarcinoma of the head and neck: preliminary report of six cases and review of the literature. Radiat Oncol 5: 89.
15. Michael H (2011) Metastasis of parotid basal cell adenocarcinoma to the hand a case report. Hand 6: 321-323.
16. Hamamoto M (2012) A case of basal cell adenocarcinoma of the parotid gland, practica oto rhino laryngological. 105: 441-446.

Part 2

Bilateral Pleomorphic Adenoma

The occurrence of multiple distinct tumors in major salivary glands is quite rare. Pleomorphic adenoma is the most common benign neoplasm of the parotid gland. However, bilateral synchronous pleomorphic adenomas occur infrequently, accounting for less than 0.2% of all parotid gland tumors (1).

Bilateral synchronous or metachronous neoplasms of the parotid gland are rarely encountered in clinical practice. The most common bilateral tumor is Warthin's tumor, with a reported incidence of 5–14%, followed by pleomorphic adenoma (2.3). Histologically, they are divided into unifocal or multifocal lesions. Even if it might be very difficult to establish, they also can be distinguished as synchronous or metachronous tumors regarding the time of their detection (3). In this part, we present a 46-year-old man with bilateral metachronous pleomorphic adenoma of the parotid gland, which was unique in the duration of the disease and the size of the mass.

II. 46-Year-Old Man with Bilateral Metachronous Pleomorphic Adenoma of the Parotid Gland

Abstract

The occurrence of multiple distinct tumors in major salivary glands is quite rare. Although the most common tumor with bilateral synchronous or metachronous development is Warthin's tumor, on rare occasions, pleomorphic adenomas have been diagnosed simultaneously as well. In this paper, we present the case of a 46-year-old man with bilateral metachronous pleomorphic adenoma of the parotid gland.

Keywords: Pleomorphic adenoma, bilateral, metachronous

Case Presentation

Clinical presentation

A 46-year-old man with a slow growing mass in the left parotid that was first diagnosed five years ago and small-sized mass in the right parotid that was diagnosed one year ago (bilateral metachronous neoplasm of the parotid gland). In palpation and bimanual examination, the mass in the left parotid gland was approximately 5 x 6cm, and it was firm and mobile without any tenderness or erythema. The facial nerve was intact (Figure 1). The mass in the right parotid gland was 3 x 2 cm, and it was firm and mobile without any inflammation. The overlying skin of mass was normal and the facial nerve had good function. There was no weight loss, sweating, or fever.

The patient did not complain of odynophagia or dysphagia. There was no bulging in the oral cavity.

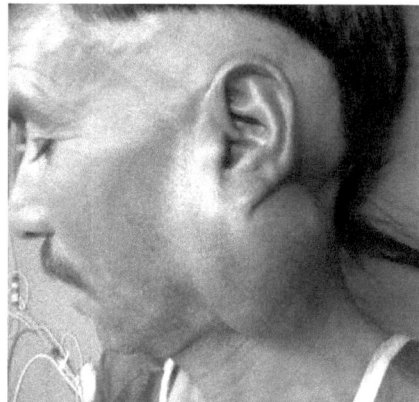

Figure1. Left side parotid Mass

Past History

The patient had no past history of cancer or infectious diseases.

Imaging

An axial CT scan showed the well-defined border of the mass in the left parotid gland with a size of 67 x 58 mm. It had solid and cystic foci with heterogeneous enhancement without any extension to stylomastoid and parapharyngeal space. On the right side, he had a well-defined, solid border mass in the right parotid with the size of 32 x 22 mm (Figure2).

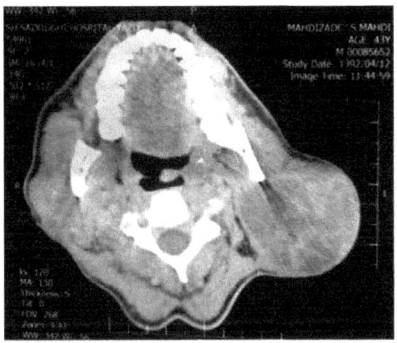

Figure2. Bilateral Parotid mass in patients, axial CT scan

Histopathology and laboratory tests

In cases of a bilateral parotid mass, systemic diseases, such as HIV, Sarcoidosis and Sjogren, should be ruled out. Sero logic tests for Sjogren syndrome, tuberculosis, cytomegalovirus, human immunodeficiency virus, and Ebstein-Barr virus were negative. FNA (fine needle aspiration) smears of right and left parotid masses showed several isolated sheets, acini of bland epithelial cells merging with the fibrillary and amorphous myxoid matrix and some bare nuclei that suggested a mixed tumor of the salivary gland (Figure 3). Permanent Pathology revealed a 7 x 5 x 5-cm mass with a creamy color and a nodular surface in the left parotid gland and a 3 x 3x 2-cm firm mass with a grayish color in the right parotid gland Microscopic Pathology showed epithelial and myoepithelial components with a chondroid background.

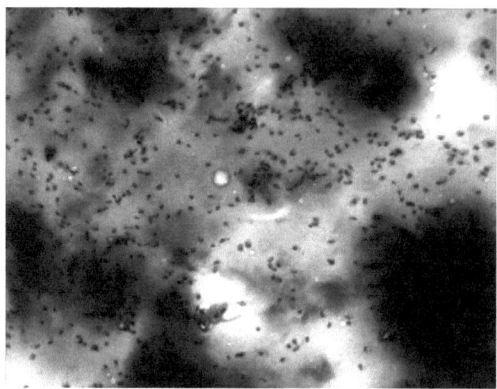

Figure3. FNA (fine needle aspiration) smears of parotid mass

Treatment and follow-up

After general anesthesia, left standard parotid incision (Blair Incision) was done, and the sub-platismal flap was elevated. Facial nerve trunk and branches were exposed and preserved and then a total parotidectomy was performed. For the right side, after facial nerve preservation, a superficial parotidectomy was performed. The facial nerve was intact, and there was no recurrence at the six-month follow-up.

Discussion

Pleomorphic adenoma, called mixed tumor because of its either epithelial and connectival component, accounts for 80% of all parotid tumors. It is mostly located at the superficial lobe of the parotid gland. The average age of onset is between 30 and 50; our case was 46.

Some authors have indicated that the mean duration of symptoms prior to diagnosis 22.9 months, with 36.5 months in male patients and 22.9 months in female patients (4). But our case had the left parotid mass for about 60 months.

Currently, according to the international literature, the most widely-used surgical procedure for the excision of a superficial lobe benign parotid tumor is superficial parotidectomy. Other inappropriate surgical treatments, such as enucleation, are strongly associated with high rates of tumor recurrence (4, 5).

The simultaneous surgical approach for parotid tumors has not been discussed extensively in the International literature. Nevertheless, some authors have stated that simultaneous parotidectomy for bilateral benign parotid glands tumours should be avoided to prevent possible bilateral facial nerve palsy (6). In 2007, C.ungari et al. (Department of Maxillofacial Surgery in Italy) indicated that bilateral pleomorphic adenoma could be surgically removed simultaneously with successful preservation of the facial nerve (7). Silva et al. from Brazil (2006) reported a patient with metachronous bilateral pleomorphic adenoma and performed total and superficial parotidectomy for the left and right tumors. However, on the left side, some facial nerve branches were removed, inducing partial paralysis (8).

Our case underwent simultaneous left total parotidectomy and right superficial parotidectomy with intact facial nerves. Thus, we would suggest simultaneous bilateral parotidectomy as the most indicated surgical approach,particularly in healthy patients with assured clinical and cytological diagnosis and without evidence of any other systemic diseases.

Conclusion

We would suggest simultaneous bilateral parotidectomy as the most indicated surgical approach, particularly in healthy patients with assured clinical and cytological diagnosis and without evidence of any other systemic disease.

References

1. Huang JT, Li W, Chen XQ. Synchronous bilateral pleomorphic adenomas of the parotid gland.J Investig Clin Dent. 2012 Aug; 3(3):225-7.

2. Toida M, Mukai K. Shimosato Y. Simultaneous occurrence of bilateral Warthin's tumors and pleomorphic adenoma in the parotid glands. J Oral Maxillofac Surg 1990 Oct; 48(10):1109-13.http://dx.doi.org/10.1016/0278-2391(90)90299-H.

3. Lefor AT, Ord RA. Multiple synchronous bilateral Warthin's tumors of the parotid glands with pleomorphic adenoma: case report and review of the literature. Oral Med Oral Pathol 1993 Sep;76(3):319-24. http://dx.doi.org/10.1016/0030- 4220(93)90260-B.

4. Junquera L, Alonso D, Sampedro A. Pleomorphic adenoma of the salivary glands: prospective clinicopa-thologic and flow cytometric study. Head Neck 1999 Oct;21(7):652-6 http://dx.doi.org/10.1002http://dx.doi.org/10.1002

5. Silva SJ, Costa Junior GT, Brant Filho AC. Metachronous bilateral pleomorphic adenoma of the parotid gland. Oral Surg Oral Med Oral Pathol Oral Radiol Endod 2006 Mar; 101(3):333-8. http://dx.doi.org/10.1016/j.tripleo.2005.07.025 PMid:16504867.

6. Turnbull AD, Frazell EL. Multiple tumors of the major salivary glands. Am J Surg 1969 Nov; 118(5):787-9.http://dx.doi.org/10.1016/0002-9610(69)90230-X.7. C. Ungari, W. Colangeli, F. Paparo, V. Bilateral Pleomorphic Adenomas Of The Parotid Glands:Discussion Over Two Cases.The Internet Journal of Head and Neck Surgery. 2007 may; 2 (1). DOI:10.5580/6c http://dx.doi.org/10.5580/6c.

8. Da Silva,G. Junior, A. Brant Filho,P. Metachronous bilateral pleomorphic adenoma of the parotid gland.Oral and Maxillofacial Pathology 2006 march;101(3): 333–8.

Part 3

Lipoma

Lipomas are among the most common benign neoplasms composed of adipose tissue. It is the most common benign form of soft tissue tumor. Many lipomas are small but can enlarge to sizes greater than several centimeters. Lipomas are commonly found in adults from 40-60 years of age, but can also be found in younger patients and children. Some authors claim that malignant transformation can occur but others refuse it. Approximately one percent of the general population has a lipoma. Lipomas are normally removed by simple excision and usually for cosmetic reasons. Lipomas are rarely observed in parotid glands. They also comprise 1–3% of all parotid neoplasms.(1) To our knowledge, lipomas in the deep lobe are extremely rare.(2)This report presents a new case of lipoma in the superficial and deep lobes of the right parotid gland.

III. Lipoma in Superficial and Deep Lobes of Parotid Gland: A Case Report

Abstract

Introduction: Lipomas among the most common benign neoplasms and rarely observed in parotid glands. We present a new case of lipoma in the superficial and deep lobes of the right parotid gland.

Case report: A 52-year-old woman with painless and progressive inflation in the right preauricular region was referred to us. Computed Tomography scanning showed a hypodense area 5.2×4 cm in dimension in the right parotid gland region, and the facial nerve was fully exposed. The patient underwent parotidectomy, during which extensive removal of the mass was done. The pathology report cited a yellow-colored fatty tissue mass, 5×4×2 in dimension. In the microscopic report, lipoma of the parotid gland was seen.

Conclusion: Determination of the exact tumor location is very important in the surgical approach in such cases. To our knowledge, this case seems to be an extremely rare case of lipoma in the superficial and deep lobes of the parotid.

Keywords: Lipoma; Parotid; Benign Tumors

Case Presentation

A 52-year-old woman with painless and progressive inflation in the right preauricular region was referred for evaluation to the ENT Department of Shahid Sadooghi Hospital in Yazd. The patient did not have any history of fever, chills, hearing problems, weight loss, and damage and infection at the site of the lesion.

On examination, the mass, 10×7 cm in dimension, was palpated at the right mandibular angle. The mass was soft, lobulated, mobile, and without pus. On oropharyngeal examination, submandibular and sublingual salivary glands, salivary secretion, nasal mucosa, and parotid duct openings were normal on both sides, and there was no obvious cervical lymphadenopathy. Computed Tomography (CT) showed a hypodense area, 5.2×4 cm in size, in the right parotid gland region (Figure 1), which originated from the superficial lobe and extended to the deep lobe with deviated lateral carotid artery branches. In addition, the facial nerve was fully exposed. The patient underwent parotidectomy, during which the inferior facial nerve branches were separated from the main mass carefully.

Furthermore, extensive removal of the mass was carried out for this patient, and the mass was sent for examination to the pathologist. The pathology report revealed a yellow-colored fatty tissue mass of 5×4×2 cm. Microscopic examination revealed adipocytes, and no malignant findings were identified (Figure2). Temporary facial nerve paralysis was seen after surgery, which disappeared completely after 2 weeks. The patient experienced no recurrence after resection for 3 months but complained of mild pain in the right jaw angle.

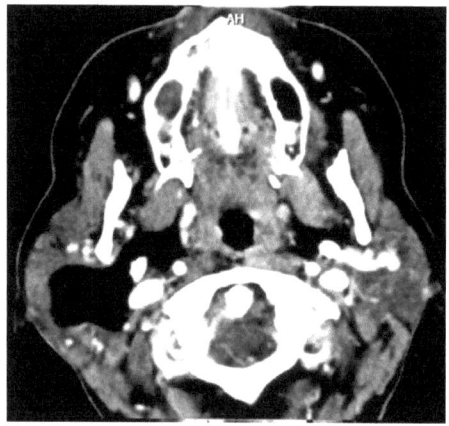

Figure1. Axial Computed Tomography scan, showing the right superficial and deep lobe parotid gland lipoma

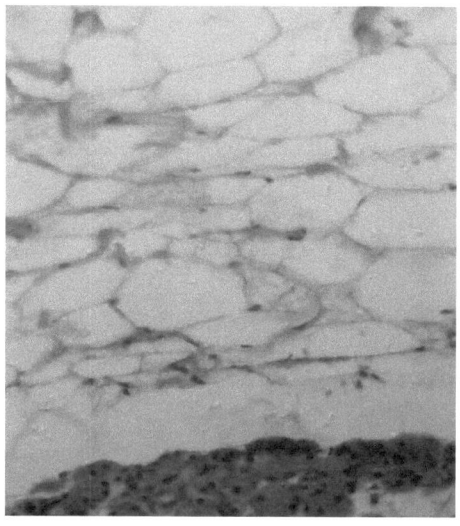

Figure2. Microscopic view of the parotid gland lipoma(Mature fat cells).

Discussion

Lipomas are rarely seen in parotid glands.(3) To the best of our knowledge, lipomas in the deep lobe are extremely rare and only 10 cases have been reported to date.(2) Because of their very low prevalence, they are often not considered as the main differential diagnosis of parotid neoplasm. What is more, lipomasin the parotid gland are very similar to mature adipose tissue histologically, and only the fibrous capsule makes them different from other fatty aggregations. (4) Lipomas in the parotid gland are often asymptomatic, but if they grow adequately, they can compress the surrounding tissue and produce an obvious tenderness. The case reported in this study had tenderness palpation on her lesion before surgery, which decreased after resection. Lipoma in this case was diagnosed first using CT scan, while in some similar studies, high-resolution CT has been advised.(5) Nevertheless, some other studies have mentioned higher accuracy of CT scan in the primary diagnosis of lipomas in the parotid glands and Magnetic Resonance Imaging (MRI) in detecting extraparotid from intraparotid lipomas.

As is mentioned in the case report, temporary facial nerve paralysis was observed after surgery.

In the previous reports, the incidence rate of facial nerve dysfunction was different from 8.2 to 65% after surgery of benign parotid tumors, and the incidence rate in lipomas in the deep lobe of the parotid was

about 80%.3 The case reported in this study underwent parotidectomy. However, surgical management of lipomas in the parotid gland is controversial, according to the surveys carried out. Some researchers recommend superficial parotidectomy, while others suggest enucleaction of well-capsulated masses.

Conclusion

In this report, a rare case of lipoma in the superficial and deep lobe of the parotid gland was reported. In such cases, determination of the exact tumor location is very important in the surgical approach. To our knowledge, this case seems to be an extremely rare case of lipoma in the superficial and deep lobe of the parotid.

References
1. Levan P, De Kerviler E, Revol M, Servant JM. Lipoma of the superficial lobe of the parotid. : a case report. Ann Chir Plast Esthet. 1997;42:333–6.
2. Chakravarti A, Dhawan R , Shashidhar T. B: Lipoma of the deep lobe of parotid gland – a case report and review of literature. Indian J. Otolaryngol. Head Neck Surg. 2008;60,194–6.
3. Cagatay Han Ulku, Yavuz Uyar. Management of lipomas arising from deep lobe of the parotid gland. Auris Nasus Larynx. 2005;32:49–53.
4. Kim YH, Reiner L. Ultrastructure of lipoma. Cancer. 1982;50:102.
5. Koreantager R, Noyek AM, Chapnik JS, Steinhardt M, Luk SC, Cooter N. Lipoma and liposarcoma of the parotid gland: high resolution preoperative imaging diagnosis. Laryngoscope. 1988;98:967–71.

Part 4

Adenoid Cystic Carcinoma

Adenoid cystic carcinoma (ACC) is generally a slow growing but highly malignant neoplasm with a remarkable capacity for recurrence. It accounted for 4.4 % of all salivary gland tumors and 11.8 % of malignant salivary gland neoplasms [1]. It affects a wide age range (9–103 years) with a peak incidence in the fifth to seventh decades, but it is very rare in children [1]. ACC commonly occurs in the major and minor salivary glands of the head and neck.

Other sites include the lungs, breasts, lacrimal glands, and skin [2].Compared to other malignancies, ACC tends to grow more slowly. Thus, patients often do well in the short-term but long-term prognosis remains guarded and most succumb to the disease within 10–15 years. Late recurrences and distant metastases remain a challenge.

Owing to the slow growth rate of the tumor, there is much controversy regarding the treatment of ACC. However, surgery remains the mainstay of management with or without radiotherapy. Distant metastasis frequently develops, mainly in the first 5 years post treatment. Local recurrences often develop even later on, warranting long term follow up of these patients. Long-term follow-up is essential regardless of the site because ACC is prone to undergo late recurrence and metastasis [3]. Most patients eventually develop distant metastases, mainly in the lungs and bone, despite the local control of the tumor. The occurrence of bone metastasis usually corresponds to rapid tumor dissemination and death of the patient, whereas lung metastases demonstrate a less aggressive clinical course [4]. The purpose of the current study is to report our experience with ACC, the relevant clinicopathological, prognostic factors and also to determine how surgical resection affect the recurrence, time of recurrence, and long-term survival of these patients.

IV. Clinicopathological Review and Survival Characteristics of Adenoid Cystic Carcinoma

Abstract

To study the clinical characters, the outcomes of treatments and the factors affecting treatment results of adenoid cystic carcinomas at Shahid Sadoughi Hospital and Shahid Ramazanzadeh radiotherapy center, Yazd, Iran.

The clinical data of 31 patients with adenoid cystic carcinoma of any anatomic site diagnosed over an 8 year period (2004–2012), were investigated retrospectively. Data regarding patients' characteristics, pathological features and follow-up were obtained from patients records. Survival rate, local recurrence and distant metastasis were analyzed using Kaplan–Meier method. Prognosis factors were analyzed by Log-rank test and Cox regression. The study included 31 patients with adenoid cystic carcinoma. The mean age at presentation was 50.2 ± 24.8 years.

There were 11 (35.5 %) males and 20 (64.5 %) females with a female predilection (M:F = 0.55:1). Parotid gland was the most common site (8/31, 25.7 %) followed by submandibular gland (7/31, 22.6 %). Perineural invasion was detected in 67.7 % of the cases. Positive surgical status was reported in 48.4 % of the specimens. Metastasis was detected in 25.8 % of the patients and the most common site of distant metastasis was lung. Overall survival rates at 2, 5, and 7 years were 95, 75, and 57 % respectively. Margin status showed significant effect on survival (P value = 0.01). Positive surgical margin is an important factor affecting the prognosis of the patients with adenoid cystic carcinoma. Surgery with negative surgical margin is the first choice of treatment for the patients with adenoid cystic carcinoma.

Our findings show that the prognosis of patients with adenoid cystic carcinoma in our center is fair.

Keywords: Adenoid cystic carcinoma, Survival, Clinicopathology

Investigation

This study was approved by the Ethics Committee of Shahid Sadoughi University of Medical Sciences. In this retrospective project, the medical records of cancer patients were reviewed from 2004 to 2012 and the medical charts of all patients diagnosed with ACC treated at Shahid Sadoughi Hospital and Shahid Ramazanzadeh Radiotherapy center, Yazd, Iran were retrieved. Variables recorded were the hospital patient registration number, date, name, age, sex, address, topography, presence or absence of perineural invasion, resection margins, node status, treatment protocol, overall survival, and time for recurrence for each subject according to the clinical data provided in their medical charts and patients follow up via phone.

Recurrence was defined as a need for additional surgery after primary tumor excision. Statistical analysis was performed with SPSS 17.0 (SPSS Inc., Chicago, IL). Survival was estimated using the Kaplan–Meier method. Univariate and multivariate logistic regression analysis was used to determine any correlation between patient-related factors and postoperative outcomes.

Results:

A total of 33 patients with ACC were treated between September 2004 and September 2012, with 31 patients meeting the necessary inclusion criteria. The age at diagnosis ranged from 18 to 99 years, with a mean age of 50.2 ± 24.8 years. There were 20 women and 11 men. The primary tumor site is given in Table 5.

Tumor site	Number	Percent
Parotid gland	8	25.7
Submandibular gland	7	22.6
Trachea	3	9.7
Bronchus	3	9.7
Maxillary sinus	3	9.7
Others	7	22.6
Sum	31	100

Table5.primary tumor site

Tumor diameter ranged 12–45 mm with a mean diameter of 24.8 ± 10 mm. Information was available regarding the state of the surgical margins at microscopic level for 26 patients, of whom 16 had tumor-free margins (51.6 %) and 10 had affected margins (48.4 %). The presence of perineural invasion (PNI) was also analyzed in 29 patients, of whom 21 (67.7 %) had microscopic PNI compared to 8 (25.8 %) who did not. 5 (19.2 %) patients had evidence of cervical lymph node metastasis at the time of diagnosis. Four (12.9 %) patients gave up surgery on initial diagnosis and 27 (87%) patients underwent primary surgical excision of their tumors. Chemotherapy was given to 4 (12.9 %) of the patients. 24 (77.4 %) of the cases had received radiotherapy. Eight (25.8 %) had evidence of distant metastasis. The most common site of distant metastasis was lung, followed by liver and bone. At the time of the study, 18 patients were alive. There were 4 deaths due to ACC, 1 death owing to unrelated cause and the remaining were lost to follow up. The average survival for our patients was 85.6 ± 8.6 months (95 % CI 68.8–102.5 months). The overall survival (OS) rates at 2, 5, 8 years were 95, 75, 57 % respectively. In the duration of 0–82 months the OS had decreased and then had not. Male patients had decreased OS compared with female patients (70.3 vs. 98.3) although this difference failed to reach statistical significance (P value = 0.21).There was no difference in OS between the age group 18–49 and 50-99 years (P value = 0.97). Survival was worse in all intervals for patients presenting with lymph node metastasis (0 % at 87 months) but again this difference failed to reach statistical significance (P value =0.73). Regarding PNI, OS in patients without PNI is longer till 45 months but after that it reaches to zero which is owing to small sample size. 48.4 % of the cases had positive surgical margin. OS in patients with positive surgical margins was 42 months less than patients with negative surgical margins (P value = 0.01). The overall recurrence rate among the patients was 33.3 % with a mean recurrence time of 65.4 months in the age group18-49 years and 60 months in the age group 50-99 years. After recurrence OS dropped until 55 months and then remained constant. There was no association between recurrence, age (P value = 0.66), gender (P value = 0.65), PNI (P value = 0.54), node metastasis (P value = 0.65) and positive surgical margin (P value = 0.42). Since majority of the patients in this study underwent radiation therapy (RT) we were unable to evaluate the relationship between OS, recurrence and RT. When the OS was compared regarding the origin of the tumor, patients with parotid, submandibular gland and bronchus tumors had the best survival (all patients were alive) and patients with trachea and maxillary sinuses tumors had the worst survival.

Discussion

This retrospective study was to evaluate the relevant clinicopathological, recurrence rate and OS in ACC patients at two institutions in Yazd, Iran. Adenoid cystic carcinoma is a rare tumor. Because of the rarity of this tumor, a small number of patients would be expected. The current study included 31 patients with ACC of any anatomic site diagnosed over an 8 year period (2004–2012). The patient population in one review was reported to range from 10 to 96 years [5]. In the current study the age at diagnosis ranged from 18 to 99 years, with a mean age of 50.2 ± 24.8 years. Gender predilection is an inconsistent feature in the literature with some authors reporting a male predominance and others finding a female or no gender predilection [6, 7]. We found a female predilection (M:F = 0.55:1). These gender differences indicate that there may be a hormonal influence accounting for biological behaviors of ACC. Up to 50 % of these tumors occur in the intraoral minor salivary glands usually in the hard palate [8]. However in the present study major salivary glands were affected more. Consistent with other study the most affected major salivary gland was the parotid gland [9]. It seems that compared to other malignancies, ACC tends to grow more slowly. Thus, patients often do well in the short-term but long-term prognosis remains guarded and most succumb to the disease within 10–15 years. Although the 5-year survival rate is high, 10- and 15-year survival markedly decreased. Hence, it is classified as ''high risk'' by the World Health Organization (WHO)[10]. The overall survival of the present study was approximately the same as, much better or less than those reported in the other studies [7, 11–14]. The differences between their data and the present study were evaluated in terms of the following: (1) the outcome for patients with ACC is site dependent [15]. In our study the majority of patients had a major salivary gland ACC which has a better outcome, likely related to surgically wider tumor-free margins, (2) it seems females had better survival outcomes, there were more females in our study (3) treatment modalities are different in different studies, (4) race might play a role, (5) the socialand economic position should not be ignored in medical behavior. Given the rare nature of this malignancy we can only attempt to identify trends; it is not possible to arrive at statistically significant conclusions. None of the variables were analyzed in relation to the survival of the disease, except for the surgical margin, showed a statistically significant relationship to it, although differences in survival can be appreciated in connection to some of these variables, such as lymph node involvement & perineural invasion. Consistent with studies by Gomez et al. [14,] and Agnes Oplatek [16] Who demonstrated decreased survival in patients with cervical nodal metastasis, our data showed a decrease in survival, too. Whereas isolated lymph node involvement without distant metastasis may not have significantly altered survival in some studies, [17] lymph node involvement is a risk factor for subsequent distant metastasis [9]. The findings of the present study are concordant with those from other study [16] confirming the important impact of tumor site at diagnosis. ACC is well known for its indolent growth but common recurrence. The overall recurrence rate among our patients was 33.3 %. The clinical course of ACC is characterized as distant metastasis; one study found that 20 % of patients developed distant metastases over the course of their follow-up [17]. Patients who were diagnosed with early-stage disease and without local recurrence of the primary tumors could also develop distant metastases [18].In one series, rate of distant metastasis was reported as 47.8 % with mean time to distant metastasis reported as approximately 5 years [19].In the current study 8 (25.8 %) patients had evidence of distant metastasis. Additionally, we did not find that increased age was associated with increased recurrence rate or overall survival which is in contrast with other study [20]. Jones et al. [21] reported that males with primary adenoid cystic carcinomas of the head and neck had a significantly better prognosis than females, while our results indicated that females had a better disease-specific survival. Consistent with other study positive surgical margin was a strong prognostic factor [9].Meanwhile, one study showed the adequacy of surgical resection did not seem to influence overall survival or recurrence rate [16]. It should be noted that a relatively high number of patients with microscopically positive margins in our and in other studies show the difficulty in determining the extension of the resection of this tumor. Furthermore, it is usually difficult for the pathologist to assess these margins in surgical specimens that are from complicated anatomical structure resections, and retraction after fixation is another problem. As a result, it is necessary to emphasize the importance of frozen section to guarantee the surgical borders of the tumor. Our study revealed that the presence of perineural invasion is associated with a decreased overall survival, although the difference was not significant. This result is in line with other study that indicates this as a negative prognostic factor [9], although there is also another study that does not find this relationship [7] which is why it is still controversial. Radical excision by surgery has been the primary treatment option. However, the extensive local infiltrative and perineural spread related to this malignancy often cause difficulty to achieve high tumor control. The effect of adjuvant radiation therapy on survival in patients with ACC is much debated. One study revealed that adjuvant radiotherapy after standard complete surgical resection was effective [22]. One recent study showed neutron radiation therapy achieved excellent 5-year local control [23]. Since majority of the patients in this study underwent RT we were unable to evaluate the relationship between OS, recurrence and RT. The role of chemotherapy for adenoid cystic carcinoma is still controversial [24].

Conclusion

ACC is relatively rare and it may result in recurrence even many years post-diagnosis. Close follow up of all patients for recurrence and metastasis is essential, although no formal guidelines exist regarding the most appropriate mode and duration of follow up. Greater knowledge of the biological behavior of these carcinomas would help us to improve the outcome of the patients. Our results showed surgery with negative surgical margin is the first choice of treatment for the patients with adenoid cystic carcinoma.

References
1. Wallace Eveson J, Nagao T (2009) Diseases of the salivary glands. In: Barnes L (ed) Surgical pathology of the head and neck, vol 1, 3rd edn. Informa Healthcare, New York, pp 552–557
2. Gondivkar SM, Gadbail AR, Chole R, Parikh RV (2011) Adenoid cystic carcinoma: a rare clinical entity and literature review. Oral Oncol 47:231–236
3. Zhao C, Liu J-Z, Wang S-C (2013) Adenoid cystic carcinoma in the maxillary gingiva: a case report and immunohistochemical study. Cancer Biol Med.10(1):52–54
4. Favia G, Maiorano E, Orsini G, Piattelli A (2000) Central (intraosseous) adenoid cystic carcinoma of the mandible: report of a case with periapical involvement. J Endod 26:760–763
5. Da Cruz Perez DE, de Abreu Alves F, Nobuko Nishimoto I, de Almeida OP, Kowalski LP (2006) Prognostic factors in head and neck adenoid cystic carcinoma. Oral Oncol 42(2):139–146
6. Triantafillidou K, Dimitrakopoulos J, Iordanidis F, Koufogiannis D (2006) Management of adenoid cystic carcinoma of minor salivary glands. J Oral Maxillofac Surg 64(7):1114–1120
7. van Weert S, Bloemena E, van der Waal I, de Bree R, Rietveld DHF, Kuik JD, René Leemans C (2013) Adenoid cystic carcinoma of the head and neck: a single-center analysis of 105consecutive cases over a 30-year period. Oral Oncol 49:824–829
8. Kumar AN, Harish M, Alavi YA, Mallikarjuna R (2013) Adenoid cystic carcinoma of buccal mucosa BMJ Case Rep. doi:10.1136/bcr-2013-009770
9. Lloyd S, Yu JB, Wilson LD, Decker RH (2011) Determinants and patterns of survival in adenoid cystic carcinoma of the head and neck, including an analysis of adjuvant radiation therapy. Am J Clin Oncol 34(1):76–81
10. Barnes L, Eveson JW, Reichart P et al (2005) World Health Organization classification of tumors: pathology and genetics. IARC, Lyon
11. Amit M, Binenbaum Y, Sharma K, Naomi DR, Ilana R, Abib A, Miles B, Yang X, Lei D, Kristine B, Christian G, Thomas M, Klaus-Dietrich W, Fliss D, Eckardt AM, Chiara C, Sesenna E, Frank P, Patel S, Gil Z (2013) Analysis of failure in patients with adenoid cystic carcinoma of the head and neck an international
collaborative study. Head Neck. 36(7):998–1004
12. Zhou Q, Chang H, Zhang H, Han Y, Liu H (2012) Increased numbers of P63-positive/CD117-positive cells in advanced adenoid cystic carcinoma give a poorer prognosis. Diagn Pathol 7:119

13. Ellington CL, Goodman M, Kono SA et al (2012) Adenoid cystic carcinoma of the head and neck. Incidence and survival trends based on 1973–2007 surveillance, epidemiology, and end results data. Cancer 118(18):4444–4451
14. Gomez DR, Hoppe BS, Wolden SL et al (2008) Outcomes and prognostic variables in adenoid cystic carcinoma of the head and neck: a recent experience. Int J Radiat Oncol Biol Phys. 70:1365–1372
15. Sengupta S, Roychowdhury A, Bandyopadhyay A (2013) Adenoid cystic carcinoma on the dorsum of the tongue. J Oral Maxillofac Pathol 17(1):98–100

16. Oplatek A, Ozer E, Agrawal A, Bapna S, Schuller DE (2010) Patterns of recurrence and survival of head and neck adenoid cystic carcinoma after definitive resection. Laryngoscope 120(1):65–70

17. Bhayani MK, Yener M, El-Naggar A, Garden A, Hanna EY, Weber RS, Kupferman ME (2012) Prognosis and risk factors for early-stage adenoid cystic carcinoma of the major salivary glands. Cancer 118(1):2872–2878

18. Gao M, Hao Y, Huang MX, Ma DQ, Luo HY, Gao Y, Peng X, Yu GY (2013) Clinicopathological study of distant metastases of salivary adenoid cystic carcinoma. Int J Oral Maxillofac Surg 42:923–928

19. Rapidis AD, Givalos N, Gakiopoulou H et al (2005) Adenoid cystic carcinoma of the head and neck: clinicopathological analysis of 23 patients and review of the literature. Oral Oncol 41(3):328–335

20. Ciccolallo L, Licitra L, Cantu' G, Gatta G (2009) Survival from salivary glands adenoid cystic carcinoma in European populations. Oral Oncol 45(8):669–674

21. Jones AS, Hamilton JW, Rowley H, Husband D, Helliwell TR (1997) Adenoid cystic carcinoma of the head and neck. Clin Otolaryngol Allied Sci 8(5):434–443

22. Elkholti Y, Cosmidis A, Ardiet JM, Laffay L, De Bari B (2013) Adenoid cystic carcinoma of the nasopharynx: a case report and a discussion about prognostic factors and the role of local treatments. Tumori 99(2):55e–60e

23. Gensheimer MF, Rainey DD, James L, Laramore JJ, Jian-Amadi GE, Chow A, Laura QM et al (2013) Neutron radiotherapy for adenoid cystic carcinoma of the lacrimal gland. Ophthalm Plast Reconstr Surg 29(4):256–260

24. Martı´nez-Rodrı´guez N, Leco-Berrocal I, Rubio-Alonso L, Arias- Irimia O, Martı´nez-Gonza´lez JM (2011) Epidemiology and treatment of adenoid cystic carcinoma of the minor salivary glands: a meta-analytic study. Med Oral Patol Oral Cir Bucal.1(16):e884–e889

Part 5

Schwannoma

More than 80 percent of parotid masses in adult patients are benign tumors. Eighty percent are pleomorphic adenomas. Schwannoma of the parotid gland is an uncommon tumor. Schwannoma rarely originates from the peripheral facial nerve or other nerves within the parotid gland. In a retrospective study, eight cases of parotid schwannoma between 1975 and 2006[1] were examined.

Facial-nerve schwannomas are uncommon. The intra-temporal portion of the nerve seems to be affected more often. Schwannomas can occur either as the result of genetic conditions, such as neurofibromatosis type I (NF1) and II (NF2), or as sporadic neoplasms[1].They are characterized by progressive facial palsy symptoms when they affect the intratemporal facial nerve. In contrast, the first symptom manifested by extratemporal schwannomas is a parotid mass, which can be mistaken with a parotid tumour[2, 3].

It is difficult to establish a correct preoperative diagnosis for facial-nerve schwannomas. It is important to suggest this diagnosis preoperatively because postoperative facial-nerve paresis or palsy is common, and these patients can be better informed of this complication before surgery[4].Although fine-needle aspiration biopsy is indicated, many of these parotid tumors are histologically defined only after or during surgery[1].

V. Schwannoma of the Parotid Gland: A Case Report

Abstract
Introduction

Schwannoma is an uncommon benign neoplasm found in the head and neck in 25-48 percent of identified cases. This tumor arises from Schwann cells and nerve sheaths. Asymptomatic swelling is the chief complaint of this tumor. Although aspiration is performed to alleviate swelling, the nature of tumor can be defined only after histopathologic examination. In fact, a schwannoma diagnosis is difficult to confirm before the surgical procedure.

Medical History

A 26-year-old woman complained of a painless mass that had been enlarging slowly in her right buccal region for five months. Five months before her presentation, she found a small mass in her right buccal region, and the mass grew larger gradually without any symptoms. She had no complaint of odynophagia, dysphagia, hoarseness, otalgia, itching,or significant weight loss. The mass was hard to the touch and mobile, with a clear boundary and no discharge, erythema in the tail of right parotid. Ultrasonography (US) revealed a hypoechoic mass 12*17*19mm in size, with irregular shape, clear boundary and no calcification.

Conclusion

The parotid gland is an uncommon location for schwannoma. There are no pathognomonic visual findings for this lesion. Only 17.6 percent of reported parotid schwannomas have been diagnosed before the surgical procedure.

FNA is not a reliable procedure for tumor diagnosis, because, in most cases, it shows a benign tumor of salivary gland i.e. pleomorphic adenoma. The nature of these tumors can be defined only after histopathologic examination. Since in histopathology of pleomorphic adenoma, myoepithelial cells were seen as schwannoma-like fusiform cells, immunohistochemistry was also performed to confirm the diagnosis. Diagnosis is confirmed with CK negative and S100 positive result

Keywords: Parotid, Schwannoma, Nouriloma

Case Presentation

A 26-year-old woman complained of a painless mass that had been enlarging slowly in her right buccal region for five months. Five month before her presentation, she found a small mass in her right buccal region, and the mass grew larger gradually without any symptoms. She had no complaint of odynophagia, dysphagia, hoarseness, otalgia, itching, or significant weight loss. Her medical history was negative.

Physical examination

The physical examination revealed a 2*2 cm mass that was hard to the touch and mobile, with a clear boundary and no discharge, erythema in the tail of right parotid.

The patient hadn't any lymphadenopathy in the supraclavicular, anterior and posterior region of the neck. The size of the mass did not change with postural changes, antibiotic therapy or eating, and no facial palsy or obstruction of the Stensen duct was present.

The clinical diagnosis was a benign tumor of the right parotid gland.

Investigation

Imaging

Routine laboratory test results were all within the reference ranges. Ultrasonography (US) revealed a hypoechoic mass 12*17*19mm in size, with irregular shape, clear boundary, and no calcification (Figure1).

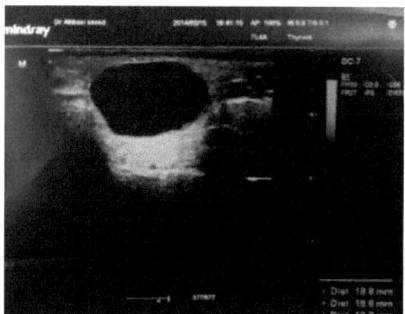

Figure1. Hypoechoic mass in right parotid gland

Treatment

Surgical resection was planned, with a standard parotid incision. During the procedure, the mass was found 1*3 cm in the superficial lobe of parotid and wasn't adhered to parotid parenchyma, Stensen duct and facial nerve. The mass was completely removed. A drain was used to remove pus, blood,and other fluid from the incision. The wound was closed tightly and healed well without complications. Histologic examination confirmed the diagnosis of parotid schwannomas.

Discussion

Schwannomas are benign tumors that arise from the nerve sheath. The estimated frequency of parotid tumors originating in the facial nerve ranges from0.2 to 1.5

percent[5].More specifically, 79 cases have been reported in the literature involving the intraparotid segment of the facial nerve[6].

The most common presenting symptom is a painless slow-growing parotid mass, and 3.9 percent of these tumors will eventually be diagnosed as malignant[7]. Preoperative diagnosis is extremely difficult due to the variation in clinical presentation and its dependency upon the nerve site involved[8]. Although facial-nerve dysfunction is generally a common symptom of facial-nerve schwannomas, it is present in only 20 percent of all cases involving the intraparotid segment[7].

Intraparotid involvement is the least common[2, 9], representing approximately 10 percent of all cases of facial nerve schwannomas[6, 10].

Preoperative diagnosis is difficult[2, 4] because FNA cytology and MRI studies are not always conclusive[6, 10, 11]. The lack of a preoperative diagnosis means that the surgeon may have to change the surgical plan based on intraoperative findings and decide what to do with a tumor that affects the facial nerve and whose resection may lead to considerable morbidity[11].

Intraoperative biopsy has also been recommended to rule out malignancy[2]but we must consider that the intraoperative diagnosis is not always correct[12].The nature of these tumors can be defined only after histopathologic examination. Since in histopathology of pleomorphic adenoma, myoepithelial cells were seen as schwannoma-like fusiform cells, immunohistochemistry was also performed to confirm the diagnosis. Diagnosis is confirmed with CK negative and S100 positive result (Figure2, 3) [13].

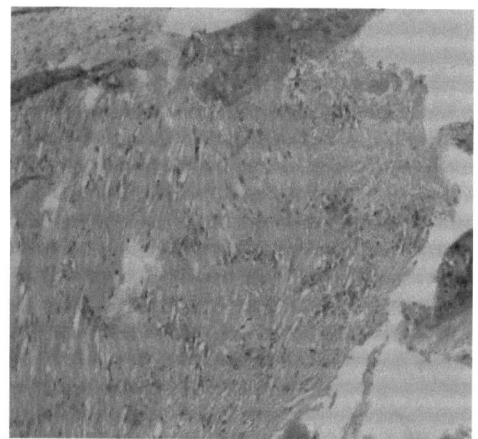

Figure2. H&E stain in parotid schwannoma

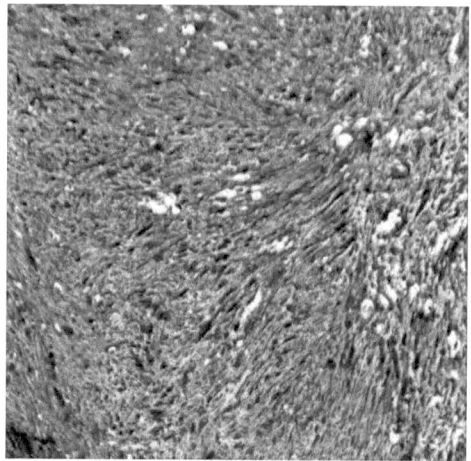

Figure3. IHC in parotid schwoannoma (S-100 positive)

Caughey et al.[5] suggested that the best indication of a schwannoma is the long course of symptoms. There are no imaging findings that can be considered as pathognomonic[14], but Shimizu et al.[4] reported that, on preoperative magnetic resonance imaging, three of five cases of facial-nerve schwannoma exhibited a target sign characterized by increased peripheral signal intensity and decreased central signal intensity on T2-weighted images. On ultrasonography, a hypoechogenic pattern with a smooth capsule can be demonstrated and guided FNA can be performed. In only 17.6 percent of the cases from the literature review did FNA cytology establish the diagnosis of aschwannoma[7]. Cytological features are quite characteristic and include fragments of spindle-shaped neoplastic cells forming Verocay bodies. Intraoperatively, inability to identify the facial nerve and the strongcohesion of the tumor with the nerve fibers are indicative of a facial-nerve schwannoma[5, 15].

References

1. Guzzo, M., et al., *Schwannoma in the parotid gland. Experience at our institute and review of the literature.* Tumori, 2009. **95**(6): p. 846-51.
2. Fyrmpas, G., et al., *Intraparotid facial nerve schwannoma: management options.* Eur Arch Otorhinolaryngol, 2008. **265**(6): p. 699-703.
3. Mehta, R.P. and D.G. Deschler, *Intraoperative diagnosis of facial nerve schwannoma at parotidectomy.* Am J Otolaryngol, 2008. **29**(2): p. 126-9.
4. Shimizu, K., et al., *Intraparotid facial nerve schwannoma: a report of five cases and an analysis of MR imaging results.* AJNR Am J Neuroradiol, 2005. **26**(6): p. 1328-30.
5. Chiang, C.W., Y.L. Chang, and P.J. Lou, *Multicentricity of intraparotid facial nerve schwannomas.* Ann Otol Rhinol Laryngol, 2001. **110**(9): p. 871-4.
6. Salemis, N.S., et al., *Large intraparotid facial nerve schwannoma: case report and review of the literature.* Int J Oral Maxillofac Surg, 2008. **37**(7): p. 679-81.
7. Marchioni, D., M. Alicandri Ciufelli, and L. Presutti, *Intraparotid facial nerve schwannoma: literature review and classification proposal.* J Laryngol Otol, 2007. **121**(8): p. 707-12.
8. Saleh, E., et al., *Facial nerve neuromas: diagnosis and management.* Am J Otol, 1995. **16**(4): p. 521-6.
9. Kumar, B.N., et al., *Intraparotid facial nerve schwannoma in a child.* J Laryngol Otol, 1996. **110**(12): p. 1169-70.
10. Kreeft, A., P.P. Schellekens, and H. Leverstein, *Intraparotid facial nerve schwannoma. What to do?* Clin Otolaryngol, 2007. **32**(2): p. 125-9.
11. Tanna, N., et al., *Intraparotid facial nerve schwannoma: clinician beware.* Ear Nose Throat J, 2009. **88**(8): p. E18-20.
12. Kang, G.C., K.C. Soo, and D.T. Lim, *Extracranial non-vestibular head and neck schwannomas: a ten-year experience.* Ann Acad Med Singapore, 2007. **36**(4): p. 233-8.
13. Moghimi M , N.M., Zarmahi S, *Schwannoma of the Parotid Gland: A Case Report.* the journal of shahid sadoughi university of medical science, 2014. **22**(3): p. 1299-1303.
14. Ginsberg, L.E. and F. DeMonte, *Diagnosis please. Case 16: facial nerve schwannoma with middle cranial fossa involvement.* Radiology, 1999. **213**(2): p. 364-8.
15. Caughey, R.J., M. May, and B.M. Schaitkin, *Intraparotid facial nerve schwannoma: diagnosis and management.* Otolaryngol Head Neck Surg, 2004. **130**(5): p. 586-92.

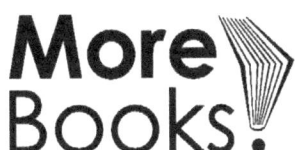
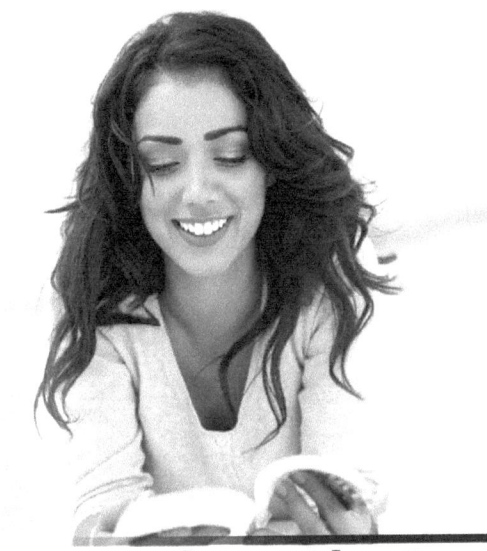
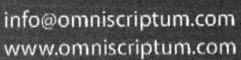
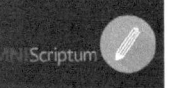

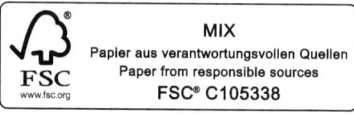

Printed by Books on Demand GmbH, Norderstedt / Germany